Blood Pressure Log

Name. _____

Date	AM		PM		
	Blood pressure	Pulse	Blood pressure	Pulse	

Level of Severity	Systolic	Diastolic
Normal	120	80
Mild Hypertension	140-160	90-100
Moderate Hypertension	160-200	100-120
Severe Hypertension	Above 200	160-200

BLOOD PRESSURE LOG

NAME. _____

Date	AM		PM		Notes
	Blood pressure	Pulse	Blood pressure	Pulse	

Level of Severity	Systolic	Diastolic
Normal	120	80
Mild Hypertension	140-160	90-100
Moderate Hypertension	160-200	100-120
Severe Hypertension	Above 200	160-200

- - - - - - - - - - - - - - - - - - - -
- - - - - - - - - - - - - - - - - - - -
- - - - - - - - - - - - - - - - - - - -
- - - - - - - - - - - - - - - - - - - -
- -
- -
- -
- -

BLOOD PRESSURE LOG

NAME. _____

Date	AM		PM		Notes
	Blood pressure	Pulse	Blood pressure	Pulse	

Level of Severity	Systolic	Diastolic
Normal	120	80
Mild Hypertension	140-160	90-100
Moderate Hypertension	160-200	100-120
Severe Hypertension	Above 200	160-200

BLOOD PRESSURE LOG

NAME. _____

Date	AM		PM		Notes
	Blood pressure	Pulse	Blood pressure	Pulse	

Level of Severity	Systolic	Diastolic
Normal	120	80
Mild Hypertension	140-160	90-100
Moderate Hypertension	160-200	100-120
Severe Hypertension	Above 200	160-200

BLOOD PRESSURE LOG

NAME. _____

Date	AM		PM		Notes
	Blood pressure	Pulse	Blood pressure	Pulse	

Level of Severity	Systolic	Diastolic
Normal	120	80
Mild Hypertension	140-160	90-100
Moderate Hypertension	160-200	100-120
Severe Hypertension	Above 200	160-200

BLOOD PRESSURE LOG

NAME. _____

Date	AM		PM		Notes
	Blood pressure	Pulse	Blood pressure	Pulse	

Level of Severity	Systolic	Diastolic
Normal	120	80
Mild Hypertension	140-160	90-100
Moderate Hypertension	160-200	100-120
Severe Hypertension	Above 200	160-200

BLOOD PRESSURE LOG

NAME. _____

Date	AM		PM		Notes
	Blood pressure	Pulse	Blood pressure	Pulse	

Level of Severity	Systolic	Diastolic
Normal	120	80
Mild Hypertension	140-160	90-100
Moderate Hypertension	160-200	100-120
Severe Hypertension	Above 200	160-200

BLOOD PRESSURE LOG

NAME. _____

Date	AM		PM		Notes
	Blood pressure	Pulse	Blood pressure	Pulse	

Level of Severity	Systolic	Diastolic
Normal	120	80
Mild Hypertension	140-160	90-100
Moderate Hypertension	160-200	100-120
Severe Hypertension	Above 200	160-200

BLOOD PRESSURE LOG

NAME. _____

Date	AM		PM		Notes
	Blood pressure	Pulse	Blood pressure	Pulse	

Level of Severity	Systolic	Diastolic
Normal	120	80
Mild Hypertension	140-160	90-100
Moderate Hypertension	160-200	100-120
Severe Hypertension	Above 200	160-200

BLOOD PRESSURE LOG

NAME. _____

Date	AM		PM		Notes
	Blood pressure	Pulse	Blood pressure	Pulse	

Level of Severity	Systolic	Diastolic
Normal	120	80
Mild Hypertension	140-160	90-100
Moderate Hypertension	160-200	100-120
Severe Hypertension	Above 200	160-200

BLOOD PRESSURE LOG

NAME. _____

Date	AM		PM		Notes
	Blood pressure	Pulse	Blood pressure	Pulse	

Level of Severity	Systolic	Diastolic
Normal	120	80
Mild Hypertension	140-160	90-100
Moderate Hypertension	160-200	100-120
Severe Hypertension	Above 200	160-200

_____
_____
_____
_____
_____
_____
_____
_____
_____
_____

BLOOD PRESSURE LOG

NAME. _____

Date	AM		PM		Notes
	Blood pressure	Pulse	Blood pressure	Pulse	

Level of Severity	Systolic	Diastolic
Normal	120	80
Mild Hypertension	140-160	90-100
Moderate Hypertension	160-200	100-120
Severe Hypertension	Above 200	160-200

BLOOD PRESSURE LOG

NAME. _____

Date	AM		PM		Notes
	Blood pressure	Pulse	Blood pressure	Pulse	

Level of Severity	Systolic	Diastolic
Normal	120	80
Mild Hypertension	140-160	90-100
Moderate Hypertension	160-200	100-120
Severe Hypertension	Above 200	160-200

BLOOD PRESSURE LOG

NAME. _____

Date	AM		PM		Notes
	Blood pressure	Pulse	Blood pressure	Pulse	

Level of Severity	Systolic	Diastolic
Normal	120	80
Mild Hypertension	140-160	90-100
Moderate Hypertension	160-200	100-120
Severe Hypertension	Above 200	160-200

BLOOD PRESSURE LOG

NAME. _____

Date	AM		PM		Notes
	Blood pressure	Pulse	Blood pressure	Pulse	

Level of Severity	Systolic	Diastolic
Normal	120	80
Mild Hypertension	140-160	90-100
Moderate Hypertension	160-200	100-120
Severe Hypertension	Above 200	160-200

BLOOD PRESSURE LOG

NAME. _____

Date	AM		PM		Notes
	Blood pressure	Pulse	Blood pressure	Pulse	

Level of Severity	Systolic	Diastolic
Normal	120	80
Mild Hypertension	140-160	90-100
Moderate Hypertension	160-200	100-120
Severe Hypertension	Above 200	160-200

BLOOD PRESSURE LOG

NAME. _____

Date	AM		PM		Notes
	Blood pressure	Pulse	Blood pressure	Pulse	

Level of Severity	Systolic	Diastolic
Normal	120	80
Mild Hypertension	140-160	90-100
Moderate Hypertension	160-200	100-120
Severe Hypertension	Above 200	160-200

BLOOD PRESSURE LOG

NAME. _____

Date	AM		PM		Notes
	Blood pressure	Pulse	Blood pressure	Pulse	

Level of Severity	Systolic	Diastolic
Normal	120	80
Mild Hypertension	140-160	90-100
Moderate Hypertension	160-200	100-120
Severe Hypertension	Above 200	160-200

BLOOD PRESSURE LOG

NAME. _____

Date	AM		PM		Notes
	Blood pressure	Pulse	Blood pressure	Pulse	

Level of Severity	Systolic	Diastolic
Normal	120	80
Mild Hypertension	140-160	90-100
Moderate Hypertension	160-200	100-120
Severe Hypertension	Above 200	160-200

BLOOD PRESSURE LOG

NAME. _____

Date	AM		PM		Notes
	Blood pressure	Pulse	Blood pressure	Pulse	

Level of Severity	Systolic	Diastolic
Normal	120	80
Mild Hypertension	140-160	90-100
Moderate Hypertension	160-200	100-120
Severe Hypertension	Above 200	160-200

BLOOD PRESSURE LOG

NAME. _____

Date	AM		PM		Notes
	Blood pressure	Pulse	Blood pressure	Pulse	

Level of Severity	Systolic	Diastolic
Normal	120	80
Mild Hypertension	140-160	90-100
Moderate Hypertension	160-200	100-120
Severe Hypertension	Above 200	160-200

BLOOD PRESSURE LOG

NAME. _____

Date	AM		PM		Notes
	Blood pressure	Pulse	Blood pressure	Pulse	

Level of Severity	Systolic	Diastolic
Normal	120	80
Mild Hypertension	140-160	90-100
Moderate Hypertension	160-200	100-120
Severe Hypertension	Above 200	160-200

BLOOD PRESSURE LOG

NAME. _____

Date	AM		PM		Notes
	Blood pressure	Pulse	Blood pressure	Pulse	

Level of Severity	Systolic	Diastolic
Normal	120	80
Mild Hypertension	140-160	90-100
Moderate Hypertension	160-200	100-120
Severe Hypertension	Above 200	160-200

BLOOD PRESSURE LOG

NAME. _____

Date	AM		PM		Notes
	Blood pressure	Pulse	Blood pressure	Pulse	

Level of Severity	Systolic	Diastolic
Normal	120	80
Mild Hypertension	140-160	90-100
Moderate Hypertension	160-200	100-120
Severe Hypertension	Above 200	160-200

BLOOD PRESSURE LOG

NAME. _____

Date	AM		PM		Notes
	Blood pressure	Pulse	Blood pressure	Pulse	

Level of Severity	Systolic	Diastolic
Normal	120	80
Mild Hypertension	140-160	90-100
Moderate Hypertension	160-200	100-120
Severe Hypertension	Above 200	160-200

BLOOD PRESSURE LOG

NAME. _____

Date	AM		PM		Notes
	Blood pressure	Pulse	Blood pressure	Pulse	

Level of Severity	Systolic	Diastolic
Normal	120	80
Mild Hypertension	140-160	90-100
Moderate Hypertension	160-200	100-120
Severe Hypertension	Above 200	160-200

BLOOD PRESSURE LOG

NAME. _____

Date	AM		PM		Notes
	Blood pressure	Pulse	Blood pressure	Pulse	

Level of Severity	Systolic	Diastolic
Normal	120	80
Mild Hypertension	140-160	90-100
Moderate Hypertension	160-200	100-120
Severe Hypertension	Above 200	160-200

BLOOD PRESSURE LOG

NAME. _____

Date	AM		PM		Notes
	Blood pressure	Pulse	Blood pressure	Pulse	

Level of Severity	Systolic	Diastolic
Normal	120	80
Mild Hypertension	140-160	90-100
Moderate Hypertension	160-200	100-120
Severe Hypertension	Above 200	160-200

BLOOD PRESSURE LOG

NAME. _____

Date	AM		PM		Notes
	Blood pressure	Pulse	Blood pressure	Pulse	

Level of Severity	Systolic	Diastolic
Normal	120	80
Mild Hypertension	140-160	90-100
Moderate Hypertension	160-200	100-120
Severe Hypertension	Above 200	160-200

BLOOD PRESSURE LOG

NAME. _____

Date	AM		PM		Notes
	Blood pressure	Pulse	Blood pressure	Pulse	

Level of Severity	Systolic	Diastolic
Normal	120	80
Mild Hypertension	140-160	90-100
Moderate Hypertension	160-200	100-120
Severe Hypertension	Above 200	160-200

BLOOD PRESSURE LOG

NAME. _____

Date	AM		PM		Notes
	Blood pressure	Pulse	Blood pressure	Pulse	

Level of Severity	Systolic	Diastolic
Normal	120	80
Mild Hypertension	140-160	90-100
Moderate Hypertension	160-200	100-120
Severe Hypertension	Above 200	160-200

BLOOD PRESSURE LOG

NAME. _____

Date	AM		PM		Notes
	Blood pressure	Pulse	Blood pressure	Pulse	

Level of Severity	Systolic	Diastolic
Normal	120	80
Mild Hypertension	140-160	90-100
Moderate Hypertension	160-200	100-120
Severe Hypertension	Above 200	160-200

BLOOD PRESSURE LOG

NAME. _____

Date	AM		PM		Notes
	Blood pressure	Pulse	Blood pressure	Pulse	

Level of Severity	Systolic	Diastolic
Normal	120	80
Mild Hypertension	140-160	90-100
Moderate Hypertension	160-200	100-120
Severe Hypertension	Above 200	160-200

BLOOD PRESSURE LOG

NAME. _____

Date	AM		PM		Notes
	Blood pressure	Pulse	Blood pressure	Pulse	

Level of Severity	Systolic	Diastolic
Normal	120	80
Mild Hypertension	140-160	90-100
Moderate Hypertension	160-200	100-120
Severe Hypertension	Above 200	160-200

BLOOD PRESSURE LOG

NAME. _____

Date	AM		PM		Notes
	Blood pressure	Pulse	Blood pressure	Pulse	

Level of Severity	Systolic	Diastolic
Normal	120	80
Mild Hypertension	140-160	90-100
Moderate Hypertension	160-200	100-120
Severe Hypertension	Above 200	160-200

BLOOD PRESSURE LOG

NAME. _____

Date	AM		PM		Notes
	Blood pressure	Pulse	Blood pressure	Pulse	

Level of Severity	Systolic	Diastolic
Normal	120	80
Mild Hypertension	140-160	90-100
Moderate Hypertension	160-200	100-120
Severe Hypertension	Above 200	160-200

BLOOD PRESSURE LOG

NAME. _____

Date	AM		PM		Notes
	Blood pressure	Pulse	Blood pressure	Pulse	

Level of Severity	Systolic	Diastolic
Normal	120	80
Mild Hypertension	140-160	90-100
Moderate Hypertension	160-200	100-120
Severe Hypertension	Above 200	160-200

BLOOD PRESSURE LOG

NAME. _____

Date	AM		PM		Notes
	Blood pressure	Pulse	Blood pressure	Pulse	

Level of Severity	Systolic	Diastolic
Normal	120	80
Mild Hypertension	140-160	90-100
Moderate Hypertension	160-200	100-120
Severe Hypertension	Above 200	160-200

BLOOD PRESSURE LOG

NAME. _____

Date	AM		PM		Notes
	Blood pressure	Pulse	Blood pressure	Pulse	

Level of Severity	Systolic	Diastolic
Normal	120	80
Mild Hypertension	140-160	90-100
Moderate Hypertension	160-200	100-120
Severe Hypertension	Above 200	160-200

BLOOD PRESSURE LOG

NAME. _____

Date	AM		PM		Notes
	Blood pressure	Pulse	Blood pressure	Pulse	

Level of Severity	Systolic	Diastolic
Normal	120	80
Mild Hypertension	140-160	90-100
Moderate Hypertension	160-200	100-120
Severe Hypertension	Above 200	160-200

BLOOD PRESSURE LOG

NAME. _____

Date	AM		PM		Notes
	Blood pressure	Pulse	Blood pressure	Pulse	

Level of Severity	Systolic	Diastolic
Normal	120	80
Mild Hypertension	140-160	90-100
Moderate Hypertension	160-200	100-120
Severe Hypertension	Above 200	160-200

BLOOD PRESSURE LOG

NAME. _____

Date	AM		PM		Notes
	Blood pressure	Pulse	Blood pressure	Pulse	

Level of Severity	Systolic	Diastolic
Normal	120	80
Mild Hypertension	140-160	90-100
Moderate Hypertension	160-200	100-120
Severe Hypertension	Above 200	160-200

BLOOD PRESSURE LOG

NAME. _____

Date	AM		PM		Notes
	Blood pressure	Pulse	Blood pressure	Pulse	

Level of Severity	Systolic	Diastolic
Normal	120	80
Mild Hypertension	140-160	90-100
Moderate Hypertension	160-200	100-120
Severe Hypertension	Above 200	160-200

BLOOD PRESSURE LOG

NAME. _____

Date	AM		PM		Notes
	Blood pressure	Pulse	Blood pressure	Pulse	

Level of Severity	Systolic	Diastolic
Normal	120	80
Mild Hypertension	140-160	90-100
Moderate Hypertension	160-200	100-120
Severe Hypertension	Above 200	160-200

BLOOD PRESSURE LOG

NAME. _____

Date	AM		PM		Notes
	Blood pressure	Pulse	Blood pressure	Pulse	

Level of Severity	Systolic	Diastolic
Normal	120	80
Mild Hypertension	140-160	90-100
Moderate Hypertension	160-200	100-120
Severe Hypertension	Above 200	160-200

BLOOD PRESSURE LOG

NAME. _____

Date	AM		PM		Notes
	Blood pressure	Pulse	Blood pressure	Pulse	

Level of Severity	Systolic	Diastolic
Normal	120	80
Mild Hypertension	140-160	90-100
Moderate Hypertension	160-200	100-120
Severe Hypertension	Above 200	160-200

BLOOD PRESSURE LOG

NAME. _____

Date	AM		PM		Notes
	Blood pressure	Pulse	Blood pressure	Pulse	

Level of Severity	Systolic	Diastolic
Normal	120	80
Mild Hypertension	140-160	90-100
Moderate Hypertension	160-200	100-120
Severe Hypertension	Above 200	160-200

BLOOD PRESSURE LOG

NAME. _____

Date	AM		PM		Notes
	Blood pressure	Pulse	Blood pressure	Pulse	

Level of Severity	Systolic	Diastolic
Normal	120	80
Mild Hypertension	140-160	90-100
Moderate Hypertension	160-200	100-120
Severe Hypertension	Above 200	160-200

BLOOD PRESSURE LOG

NAME. _____

Date	AM		PM		Notes
	Blood pressure	Pulse	Blood pressure	Pulse	

Level of Severity	Systolic	Diastolic
Normal	120	80
Mild Hypertension	140-160	90-100
Moderate Hypertension	160-200	100-120
Severe Hypertension	Above 200	160-200

BLOOD PRESSURE LOG

NAME. _____

Date	AM		PM		Notes
	Blood pressure	Pulse	Blood pressure	Pulse	

Level of Severity	Systolic	Diastolic
Normal	120	80
Mild Hypertension	140-160	90-100
Moderate Hypertension	160-200	100-120
Severe Hypertension	Above 200	160-200

Blood Pressure Log

Name. _____

Date	AM		PM		Notes
	Blood pressure	Pulse	Blood pressure	Pulse	

Level of Severity	Systolic	Diastolic
Normal	120	80
Mild Hypertension	140-160	90-100
Moderate Hypertension	160-200	100-120
Severe Hypertension	Above 200	160-200

BLOOD PRESSURE LOG

NAME. _____

Date	AM		PM		Notes
	Blood pressure	Pulse	Blood pressure	Pulse	

Level of Severity	Systolic	Diastolic
Normal	120	80
Mild Hypertension	140-160	90-100
Moderate Hypertension	160-200	100-120
Severe Hypertension	Above 200	160-200

BLOOD PRESSURE LOG

NAME. _____

Date	AM		PM		Notes
	Blood pressure	Pulse	Blood pressure	Pulse	

Level of Severity	Systolic	Diastolic
Normal	120	80
Mild Hypertension	140-160	90-100
Moderate Hypertension	160-200	100-120
Severe Hypertension	Above 200	160-200

BLOOD PRESSURE LOG

NAME. _____

Date	AM		PM		Notes
	Blood pressure	Pulse	Blood pressure	Pulse	

Level of Severity	Systolic	Diastolic
Normal	120	80
Mild Hypertension	140-160	90-100
Moderate Hypertension	160-200	100-120
Severe Hypertension	Above 200	160-200

BLOOD PRESSURE LOG

NAME. _____

Date	AM		PM		Notes
	Blood pressure	Pulse	Blood pressure	Pulse	

Level of Severity	Systolic	Diastolic
Normal	120	80
Mild Hypertension	140-160	90-100
Moderate Hypertension	160-200	100-120
Severe Hypertension	Above 200	160-200

BLOOD PRESSURE LOG

NAME. _____

Date	AM		PM		Notes
	Blood pressure	Pulse	Blood pressure	Pulse	

Level of Severity	Systolic	Diastolic
Normal	120	80
Mild Hypertension	140-160	90-100
Moderate Hypertension	160-200	100-120
Severe Hypertension	Above 200	160-200

BLOOD PRESSURE LOG

NAME. _____

Date	AM		PM		Notes
	Blood pressure	Pulse	Blood pressure	Pulse	

Level of Severity	Systolic	Diastolic
Normal	120	80
Mild Hypertension	140-160	90-100
Moderate Hypertension	160-200	100-120
Severe Hypertension	Above 200	160-200

BLOOD PRESSURE LOG

NAME. _____

Date	AM		PM		Notes
	Blood pressure	Pulse	Blood pressure	Pulse	

Level of Severity	Systolic	Diastolic
Normal	120	80
Mild Hypertension	140-160	90-100
Moderate Hypertension	160-200	100-120
Severe Hypertension	Above 200	160-200

BLOOD PRESSURE LOG

NAME. _____

Date	AM		PM		Notes
	Blood pressure	Pulse	Blood pressure	Pulse	

Level of Severity	Systolic	Diastolic
Normal	120	80
Mild Hypertension	140-160	90-100
Moderate Hypertension	160-200	100-120
Severe Hypertension	Above 200	160-200

BLOOD PRESSURE LOG

NAME. _____

Date	AM		PM		Notes
	Blood pressure	Pulse	Blood pressure	Pulse	

Level of Severity	Systolic	Diastolic
Normal	120	80
Mild Hypertension	140-160	90-100
Moderate Hypertension	160-200	100-120
Severe Hypertension	Above 200	160-200

BLOOD PRESSURE LOG

NAME. _____

Date	AM		PM		Notes
	Blood pressure	Pulse	Blood pressure	Pulse	

Level of Severity	Systolic	Diastolic
Normal	120	80
Mild Hypertension	140-160	90-100
Moderate Hypertension	160-200	100-120
Severe Hypertension	Above 200	160-200

BLOOD PRESSURE LOG

NAME. _____

Date	AM		PM		Notes
	Blood pressure	Pulse	Blood pressure	Pulse	

Level of Severity	Systolic	Diastolic
Normal	120	80
Mild Hypertension	140-160	90-100
Moderate Hypertension	160-200	100-120
Severe Hypertension	Above 200	160-200

BLOOD PRESSURE LOG

NAME. _____

Date	AM		PM		Notes
	Blood pressure	Pulse	Blood pressure	Pulse	

Level of Severity	Systolic	Diastolic
Normal	120	80
Mild Hypertension	140-160	90-100
Moderate Hypertension	160-200	100-120
Severe Hypertension	Above 200	160-200

BLOOD PRESSURE LOG

NAME. _____

Date	AM		PM		Notes
	Blood pressure	Pulse	Blood pressure	Pulse	

Level of Severity	Systolic	Diastolic
Normal	120	80
Mild Hypertension	140-160	90-100
Moderate Hypertension	160-200	100-120
Severe Hypertension	Above 200	160-200

BLOOD PRESSURE LOG

NAME. _____

Date	AM		PM		Notes
	Blood pressure	Pulse	Blood pressure	Pulse	

Level of Severity	Systolic	Diastolic
Normal	120	80
Mild Hypertension	140-160	90-100
Moderate Hypertension	160-200	100-120
Severe Hypertension	Above 200	160-200

BLOOD PRESSURE LOG

NAME. _____

Date	AM		PM		Notes
	Blood pressure	Pulse	Blood pressure	Pulse	

Level of Severity	Systolic	Diastolic
Normal	120	80
Mild Hypertension	140-160	90-100
Moderate Hypertension	160-200	100-120
Severe Hypertension	Above 200	160-200

BLOOD PRESSURE LOG

NAME. _____

Date	AM		PM		Notes
	Blood pressure	Pulse	Blood pressure	Pulse	

Level of Severity	Systolic	Diastolic
Normal	120	80
Mild Hypertension	140-160	90-100
Moderate Hypertension	160-200	100-120
Severe Hypertension	Above 200	160-200

_____
_____
_____
_____
_____
_____
_____
_____
_____

Blood Pressure Log

Name. _____

Date	AM		PM		Notes
	Blood pressure	Pulse	Blood pressure	Pulse	

Level of Severity	Systolic	Diastolic
Normal	120	80
Mild Hypertension	140-160	90-100
Moderate Hypertension	160-200	100-120
Severe Hypertension	Above 200	160-200

BLOOD PRESSURE LOG

NAME. _____

Date	AM		PM		Notes
	Blood pressure	Pulse	Blood pressure	Pulse	

Level of Severity	Systolic	Diastolic
Normal	120	80
Mild Hypertension	140-160	90-100
Moderate Hypertension	160-200	100-120
Severe Hypertension	Above 200	160-200

BLOOD PRESSURE LOG

NAME. _____

Date	AM		PM		Notes
	Blood pressure	Pulse	Blood pressure	Pulse	

Level of Severity	Systolic	Diastolic
Normal	120	80
Mild Hypertension	140-160	90-100
Moderate Hypertension	160-200	100-120
Severe Hypertension	Above 200	160-200

BLOOD PRESSURE LOG

NAME. _____

Date	AM		PM		Notes
	Blood pressure	Pulse	Blood pressure	Pulse	

Level of Severity	Systolic	Diastolic
Normal	120	80
Mild Hypertension	140-160	90-100
Moderate Hypertension	160-200	100-120
Severe Hypertension	Above 200	160-200

BLOOD PRESSURE LOG

NAME. _____

Date	AM		PM		Notes
	Blood pressure	Pulse	Blood pressure	Pulse	

Level of Severity	Systolic	Diastolic
Normal	120	80
Mild Hypertension	140-160	90-100
Moderate Hypertension	160-200	100-120
Severe Hypertension	Above 200	160-200

BLOOD PRESSURE LOG

NAME. _____

Date	AM		PM		Notes
	Blood pressure	Pulse	Blood pressure	Pulse	

Level of Severity	Systolic	Diastolic
Normal	120	80
Mild Hypertension	140-160	90-100
Moderate Hypertension	160-200	100-120
Severe Hypertension	Above 200	160-200

BLOOD PRESSURE LOG

NAME. _____

Date	AM		PM		Notes
	Blood pressure	Pulse	Blood pressure	Pulse	

Level of Severity	Systolic	Diastolic
Normal	120	80
Mild Hypertension	140-160	90-100
Moderate Hypertension	160-200	100-120
Severe Hypertension	Above 200	160-200

BLOOD PRESSURE LOG

NAME. _____

Date	AM		PM		Notes
	Blood pressure	Pulse	Blood pressure	Pulse	

Level of Severity	Systolic	Diastolic
Normal	120	80
Mild Hypertension	140-160	90-100
Moderate Hypertension	160-200	100-120
Severe Hypertension	Above 200	160-200

BLOOD PRESSURE LOG

NAME. _____

Date	AM		PM		Notes
	Blood pressure	Pulse	Blood pressure	Pulse	

Level of Severity	Systolic	Diastolic
Normal	120	80
Mild Hypertension	140-160	90-100
Moderate Hypertension	160-200	100-120
Severe Hypertension	Above 200	160-200

BLOOD PRESSURE LOG

NAME. _____

Date	AM		PM		Notes
	Blood pressure	Pulse	Blood pressure	Pulse	

Level of Severity	Systolic	Diastolic
Normal	120	80
Mild Hypertension	140-160	90-100
Moderate Hypertension	160-200	100-120
Severe Hypertension	Above 200	160-200

BLOOD PRESSURE LOG

NAME. _____

Date	AM		PM		Notes
	Blood pressure	Pulse	Blood pressure	Pulse	

Level of Severity	Systolic	Diastolic
Normal	120	80
Mild Hypertension	140-160	90-100
Moderate Hypertension	160-200	100-120
Severe Hypertension	Above 200	160-200

BLOOD PRESSURE LOG

NAME. _____

Date	AM		PM		Notes
	Blood pressure	Pulse	Blood pressure	Pulse	

Level of Severity	Systolic	Diastolic
Normal	120	80
Mild Hypertension	140-160	90-100
Moderate Hypertension	160-200	100-120
Severe Hypertension	Above 200	160-200

BLOOD PRESSURE LOG

NAME. _____

Date	AM		PM		Notes
	Blood pressure	Pulse	Blood pressure	Pulse	

Level of Severity	Systolic	Diastolic
Normal	120	80
Mild Hypertension	140-160	90-100
Moderate Hypertension	160-200	100-120
Severe Hypertension	Above 200	160-200

BLOOD PRESSURE LOG

NAME. _____

Date	AM		PM		Notes
	Blood pressure	Pulse	Blood pressure	Pulse	

Level of Severity	Systolic	Diastolic
Normal	120	80
Mild Hypertension	140-160	90-100
Moderate Hypertension	160-200	100-120
Severe Hypertension	Above 200	160-200

BLOOD PRESSURE LOG

NAME. _____

Date	AM		PM		Notes
	Blood pressure	Pulse	Blood pressure	Pulse	

Level of Severity	Systolic	Diastolic
Normal	120	80
Mild Hypertension	140-160	90-100
Moderate Hypertension	160-200	100-120
Severe Hypertension	Above 200	160-200

Blood Pressure Log

Name. _____

Date	AM		PM		Notes
	Blood pressure	Pulse	Blood pressure	Pulse	

Level of Severity	Systolic	Diastolic
Normal	120	80
Mild Hypertension	140-160	90-100
Moderate Hypertension	160-200	100-120
Severe Hypertension	Above 200	160-200

BLOOD PRESSURE LOG

NAME. _____

Date	AM		PM		Notes
	Blood pressure	Pulse	Blood pressure	Pulse	

Level of Severity	Systolic	Diastolic
Normal	120	80
Mild Hypertension	140-160	90-100
Moderate Hypertension	160-200	100-120
Severe Hypertension	Above 200	160-200

BLOOD PRESSURE LOG

NAME. _____

Date	AM		PM		Notes
	Blood pressure	Pulse	Blood pressure	Pulse	

Level of Severity	Systolic	Diastolic
Normal	120	80
Mild Hypertension	140-160	90-100
Moderate Hypertension	160-200	100-120
Severe Hypertension	Above 200	160-200

BLOOD PRESSURE LOG

NAME. _____

Date	AM		PM		Notes
	Blood pressure	Pulse	Blood pressure	Pulse	

Level of Severity	Systolic	Diastolic
Normal	120	80
Mild Hypertension	140-160	90-100
Moderate Hypertension	160-200	100-120
Severe Hypertension	Above 200	160-200

BLOOD PRESSURE LOG

NAME. _____

Date	AM		PM		Notes
	Blood pressure	Pulse	Blood pressure	Pulse	

Level of Severity	Systolic	Diastolic
Normal	120	80
Mild Hypertension	140-160	90-100
Moderate Hypertension	160-200	100-120
Severe Hypertension	Above 200	160-200

BLOOD PRESSURE LOG

NAME. _____

Date	AM		PM		Notes
	Blood pressure	Pulse	Blood pressure	Pulse	

Level of Severity	Systolic	Diastolic
Normal	120	80
Mild Hypertension	140-160	90-100
Moderate Hypertension	160-200	100-120
Severe Hypertension	Above 200	160-200

BLOOD PRESSURE LOG

NAME. _____

Date	AM		PM		Notes
	Blood pressure	Pulse	Blood pressure	Pulse	

Level of Severity	Systolic	Diastolic
Normal	120	80
Mild Hypertension	140-160	90-100
Moderate Hypertension	160-200	100-120
Severe Hypertension	Above 200	160-200

BLOOD PRESSURE LOG

NAME. _____

Date	AM		PM		Notes
	Blood pressure	Pulse	Blood pressure	Pulse	

Level of Severity	Systolic	Diastolic
Normal	120	80
Mild Hypertension	140-160	90-100
Moderate Hypertension	160-200	100-120
Severe Hypertension	Above 200	160-200

BLOOD PRESSURE LOG

NAME. _____

Date	AM		PM		Notes
	Blood pressure	Pulse	Blood pressure	Pulse	

Level of Severity	Systolic	Diastolic
Normal	120	80
Mild Hypertension	140-160	90-100
Moderate Hypertension	160-200	100-120
Severe Hypertension	Above 200	160-200

BLOOD PRESSURE LOG

NAME. _____

Date	AM		PM		Notes
	Blood pressure	Pulse	Blood pressure	Pulse	

Level of Severity	Systolic	Diastolic
Normal	120	80
Mild Hypertension	140-160	90-100
Moderate Hypertension	160-200	100-120
Severe Hypertension	Above 200	160-200

BLOOD PRESSURE LOG

NAME. _____

Date	AM		PM		Notes
	Blood pressure	Pulse	Blood pressure	Pulse	

Level of Severity	Systolic	Diastolic
Normal	120	80
Mild Hypertension	140-160	90-100
Moderate Hypertension	160-200	100-120
Severe Hypertension	Above 200	160-200

BLOOD PRESSURE LOG

NAME. _____

Date	AM		PM		Notes
	Blood pressure	Pulse	Blood pressure	Pulse	

Level of Severity	Systolic	Diastolic
Normal	120	80
Mild Hypertension	140-160	90-100
Moderate Hypertension	160-200	100-120
Severe Hypertension	Above 200	160-200

BLOOD PRESSURE LOG

NAME. _____

Date	AM		PM		Notes
	Blood pressure	Pulse	Blood pressure	Pulse	

Level of Severity	Systolic	Diastolic
Normal	120	80
Mild Hypertension	140-160	90-100
Moderate Hypertension	160-200	100-120
Severe Hypertension	Above 200	160-200

BLOOD PRESSURE LOG

NAME. _____

| Date | AM | | PM | | Notes |
	Blood pressure	Pulse	Blood pressure	Pulse	

Level of Severity	Systolic	Diastolic
Normal	120	80
Mild Hypertension	140-160	90-100
Moderate Hypertension	160-200	100-120
Severe Hypertension	Above 200	160-200

BLOOD PRESSURE LOG

NAME. _____

Date	AM		PM		Notes
	Blood pressure	Pulse	Blood pressure	Pulse	

Level of Severity	Systolic	Diastolic
Normal	120	80
Mild Hypertension	140-160	90-100
Moderate Hypertension	160-200	100-120
Severe Hypertension	Above 200	160-200

BLOOD PRESSURE LOG

NAME. _____

Date	AM		PM		Notes
	Blood pressure	Pulse	Blood pressure	Pulse	

Level of Severity	Systolic	Diastolic
Normal	120	80
Mild Hypertension	140-160	90-100
Moderate Hypertension	160-200	100-120
Severe Hypertension	Above 200	160-200

BLOOD PRESSURE LOG

NAME. _____

Date	AM		PM		Notes
	Blood pressure	Pulse	Blood pressure	Pulse	

Level of Severity	Systolic	Diastolic
Normal	120	80
Mild Hypertension	140-160	90-100
Moderate Hypertension	160-200	100-120
Severe Hypertension	Above 200	160-200

_____
_____
_____
_____
_____
_____
_____
_____
_____
_____

BLOOD PRESSURE LOG

NAME. _____

Date	AM		PM		Notes
	Blood pressure	Pulse	Blood pressure	Pulse	

Level of Severity	Systolic	Diastolic
Normal	120	80
Mild Hypertension	140-160	90-100
Moderate Hypertension	160-200	100-120
Severe Hypertension	Above 200	160-200

BLOOD PRESSURE LOG

NAME. _____

Date	AM		PM		Notes
	Blood pressure	Pulse	Blood pressure	Pulse	

Level of Severity	Systolic	Diastolic
Normal	120	80
Mild Hypertension	140-160	90-100
Moderate Hypertension	160-200	100-120
Severe Hypertension	Above 200	160-200

BLOOD PRESSURE LOG

NAME. _____

Date	AM		PM		Notes
	Blood pressure	Pulse	Blood pressure	Pulse	

Level of Severity	Systolic	Diastolic
Normal	120	80
Mild Hypertension	140-160	90-100
Moderate Hypertension	160-200	100-120
Severe Hypertension	Above 200	160-200

BLOOD PRESSURE LOG

NAME. _____

Date	AM		PM		Notes
	Blood pressure	Pulse	Blood pressure	Pulse	

Level of Severity	Systolic	Diastolic
Normal	120	80
Mild Hypertension	140-160	90-100
Moderate Hypertension	160-200	100-120
Severe Hypertension	Above 200	160-200

Blood Pressure Log

Name. _____

Date	AM		PM		Notes
	Blood pressure	Pulse	Blood pressure	Pulse	

Level of Severity	Systolic	Diastolic
Normal	120	80
Mild Hypertension	140-160	90-100
Moderate Hypertension	160-200	100-120
Severe Hypertension	Above 200	160-200

BLOOD PRESSURE LOG

NAME. _____

Date	AM		PM		Notes
	Blood pressure	Pulse	Blood pressure	Pulse	

Level of Severity	Systolic	Diastolic
Normal	120	80
Mild Hypertension	140-160	90-100
Moderate Hypertension	160-200	100-120
Severe Hypertension	Above 200	160-200

BLOOD PRESSURE LOG

NAME. _____

Date	AM		PM		Notes
	Blood pressure	Pulse	Blood pressure	Pulse	

Level of Severity	Systolic	Diastolic
Normal	120	80
Mild Hypertension	140-160	90-100
Moderate Hypertension	160-200	100-120
Severe Hypertension	Above 200	160-200

BLOOD PRESSURE LOG

NAME. _____

Date	AM		PM		Notes
	Blood pressure	Pulse	Blood pressure	Pulse	

Level of Severity	Systolic	Diastolic
Normal	120	80
Mild Hypertension	140-160	90-100
Moderate Hypertension	160-200	100-120
Severe Hypertension	Above 200	160-200

Blood Pressure Log

NAME. _____

Date	AM		PM		Notes
	Blood pressure	Pulse	Blood pressure	Pulse	

Level of Severity	Systolic	Diastolic
Normal	120	80
Mild Hypertension	140-160	90-100
Moderate Hypertension	160-200	100-120
Severe Hypertension	Above 200	160-200

BLOOD PRESSURE LOG

NAME. _____

Date	AM		PM		Notes
	Blood pressure	Pulse	Blood pressure	Pulse	

Level of Severity	Systolic	Diastolic
Normal	120	80
Mild Hypertension	140-160	90-100
Moderate Hypertension	160-200	100-120
Severe Hypertension	Above 200	160-200

BLOOD PRESSURE LOG

NAME. _____

Date	AM		PM		Notes
	Blood pressure	Pulse	Blood pressure	Pulse	

Level of Severity	Systolic	Diastolic
Normal	120	80
Mild Hypertension	140-160	90-100
Moderate Hypertension	160-200	100-120
Severe Hypertension	Above 200	160-200

www.ingramcontent.com/pod-product-compliance
Lightning Source LLC
Chambersburg PA
CBHW072101280526
45788CB00006B/2355